Heart healthy diet

Meal plans and shopping guide to deal with heart problems

Robert Berry

Table of contents

Introduction. 5

Chapter 1. 11

Understanding the Importance of Heart Health

Chapter 2. 20

Nutritional Guidelines for a Heart Healthy Diet

Chapter 3. 72

Planning Your Heart Healthy Meals

Chapter 4. 95

Staying Hydrated and Limiting

Alcohol Consumption

Chapter 5. 106

Reducing Stress and Incorporating

Physical Activity

Chapter 6. 115

Healthy Cooking Techniques for

Heart Health

Chapter 7. 123

Sample Meal Plans and Recipes for a

Heart Healthy Diet

Chapter 8. 133

Special Considerations for

Individuals with Specific Heart
Conditions

Chapter 9. 146

Tips for Dining Out and Traveling on
a Heart Healthy Diet

Conclusion. 155

Introduction.

In our fast-paced world today, it can be challenging to prioritize our health. We often find ourselves rushing through meals, grabbing quick snacks, and neglecting the importance of a balanced diet. As a result, heart disease has become one of the leading causes of death worldwide, highlighting the urgent need for lifestyle changes that promote heart health.

This book aims to empower you with the knowledge and tools to adopt a heart-healthy diet, making conscious decisions that nourish your most vital organ. Whether you are seeking to prevent heart disease, manage a current condition, or simply improve your overall well-being, this comprehensive guide will serve as your compass towards a healthier lifestyle.

Within these pages, you will find a wealth of information about the benefits of a heart-healthy diet, including its impact on your cardiovascular health, weight management, and overall longevity. Together, we will explore the fundamental principles of nutrition and delve into the intricate mechanisms that underlie heart disease. Armed with this knowledge, you will be better equipped to make informed choices about the foods you consume, while still savoring delicious and satisfying meals.

This book goes beyond merely outlining dietary guidelines; it provides you with practical tips, expert advice, and mouthwatering recipes that will make your transition to a heart-healthy lifestyle seamless and enjoyable. You will learn how to navigate the grocery store, decipher nutrition labels, and incorporate a variety of heart-boosting ingredients into your meals. Furthermore, we will address common misconceptions surrounding popular diets and shed light on the most effective strategies for sustaining long-term success.

While diet plays a crucial role in heart health, we cannot overlook the significance of exercise and stress management. Therefore, this book features an exploration of various physical activities, relaxation techniques, and mindfulness practices that complement your dietary choices, promoting a holistic approach to cardiovascular wellness.

The journey to better heart health may seem daunting, but with the guidance and support provided here, you will discover that it is an exciting path filled with delicious meals, newfound energy, and a sense of vitality. So, let us begin this transformative journey together as we embark upon a heart-healthy diet that will improve not only our cardiovascular health but also enrich our overall quality of life.

Chapter 1.

Understanding the Importance of Heart Health

The human heart is a magnificent organ that beats tirelessly throughout our lives, pumping life-giving oxygenated blood to every cell in our bodies. Despite its vital role in sustaining our lives, many of us take our heart's health for granted. In this chapter, we will delve into the significance of heart health, exploring how it impacts our overall well-being and quality of life. We'll also discuss strategies to maintain a healthy heart and prevent cardiovascular diseases.

The Heart's Anatomy and Function

Before diving into the importance of heart health, let's understand the anatomy and function of our hearts. The heart consists of four chambers: the two upper chambers called atria, and the two lower chambers known as ventricles. Its primary function is to circulate blood through a vast network of blood vessels, ensuring that every part of our body receives the necessary nutrients and oxygen.

The Journey: Understanding Cardiovascular diseases

Cardiovascular diseases (CVDs) encompass a range of conditions that affect the heart and blood vessels. These diseases include coronary artery disease, heart failure, arrhythmias, and stroke, accounting for a significant portion of global mortality. Understanding the risk factors leading to CVDs is crucial in appreciating the importance of heart health.

The Impact of Heart Health on

Quality of Life

Maintaining a healthy heart has a profound impact on our overall well-being and quality of life. A healthy heart means efficient blood circulation, leading to better oxygenation, reduced fatigue, and improved stamina. It also lowers the risk of developing debilitating conditions such as heart attacks, strokes, and heart failure, which can significantly impact our physical and emotional state.

Preventing the Silent Killer: Heart

Disease

Coronary artery disease is a leading cause of heart attacks, which often strike without warning. The importance of heart health in preventing heart disease cannot be overstated. Adopting a heart-healthy lifestyle can significantly reduce the risk factors, such as hypertension, high cholesterol levels, and obesity. Regular exercise, a nutritious diet, stress management, and avoiding tobacco products are key components in maintaining a healthy heart and preventing cardiac issues.

Detecting and Treating Heart Conditions

Early detection and treatment of heart conditions play a vital role in preserving heart health. Routine check-ups, incorporating regular blood pressure monitoring and cholesterol level assessments, enable healthcare professionals to identify potential problems before they escalate. Moreover, advances in medical technology have brought about various diagnostic tests and treatment options, ranging from medication to surgical interventions, allowing us to address heart-related issues effectively.

Improving Heart Health through Lifestyle Modifications

A heart-healthy lifestyle is built on several key principles that can improve heart health and overall well-being. Regular physical activity, such as aerobic exercises, strengthens the heart muscles and improves overall cardiovascular fitness. A well-balanced diet, rich in fruits, vegetables, lean proteins, and whole grains, provides the necessary nutrients while reducing the intake of unhealthy fats, sodium, and added sugars. Managing stress, practicing mindfulness, and getting enough sleep are equally important in maintaining heart health.

Understanding the importance of heart health encompasses recognizing the intricate role our hearts play in our daily lives. By valuing our heart's well-being, adopting preventive measures, and being proactive about regular screenings, we can maintain optimal heart health. Through small changes to our lifestyle and prioritizing heart-healthy habits, we hold the power to protect our hearts and ensure a longer, healthier life.

Chapter 2

Nutritional Guidelines for a Heart Healthy Diet

2.1. Limiting Saturated and Trans Fats

Maintaining a heart-healthy diet is essential for reducing the risk of cardiovascular diseases. One crucial aspect of such a diet is the careful management of saturated and trans fats intake. These two types of fats are known to raise cholesterol levels, particularly LDL cholesterol, which can clog arteries and lead to heart disease. By limiting the consumption of saturated and trans fats, individuals can significantly improve their heart health.

Saturated fats are primarily found in animal products such as red meat, poultry, and full-fat dairy products. They are also present in certain plant-based oils like coconut oil and palm oil. While it's not necessary to completely eliminate saturated fats from the diet, it's important to consume them in moderation.

Healthier options for cooking and flavoring foods include olive oil, canola oil, and avocado oil, which are rich in monounsaturated and polyunsaturated fats that can actually help lower LDL cholesterol levels.

Trans fats, on the other hand, are commonly found in processed and packaged foods such as cookies, crackers, and fried foods. These artificial fats are created through a process called hydrogenation, which turns liquid oils into solid fats to extend the shelf life of food products. However, trans fats have been shown to raise LDL cholesterol and lower HDL cholesterol, making them especially detrimental to heart health. In many countries, there are restrictions and bans on the use of trans fats in food production, but it's still important for consumers to check food labels and avoid products containing partially hydrogenated oils.

To limit the intake of saturated and

trans fats, individuals can make simple yet impactful changes to their diet. Choosing lean cuts of meat, trimming visible fat from meat, and opting for skinless poultry can reduce saturated fat intake. Additionally, selecting low-fat or fat-free dairy products can help minimize the consumption of saturated fats. When it comes to trans fats, reading food labels is crucial. Avoiding products that list "partially hydrogenated oils" in the ingredient list is a surefire way to steer clear of trans fats.

Incorporating heart-healthy fats such as those found in nuts, seeds, and fatty fish like salmon and mackerel can further improve the overall lipid profile and promote heart health. These sources of unsaturated fats contain omega-3 fatty acids, which have been shown to reduce the risk of heart disease.

In conclusion, limiting saturated and trans fats is an important aspect of a healthy heart diet. By being mindful of food choices and opting for healthier fats, individuals can make significant strides in protecting their cardiovascular health. Making small, sustainable changes to reduce saturated and trans fats in the diet can contribute to long-term heart health and overall well-being.

2.2. Increasing Intake of Omega-3 Fatty Acids

Omega-3 fatty acids are essential fats that play a crucial role in maintaining heart health. They are known for their ability to reduce inflammation, lower blood triglyceride levels, and decrease the risk of developing heart disease. Incorporating omega-3 fatty acids into one's diet can have a significant positive impact on overall cardiovascular well-being.

There are three main types of omega -3 fatty acids: alpha-linolenic acid (ALA), eicosapentaenoic acid (EPA), and docosahexaenoic acid (DHA). ALA is primarily found in plant-based sources such as flaxseeds, chia seeds, and walnuts. EPA and DHA, on the other hand, are predominantly found in fatty fish like salmon, mackerel, and sardines. While ALA is beneficial, EPA and DHA are particularly potent in promoting heart health.

One of the most well-established benefits of omega-3 fatty acids is their ability to reduce the risk of arrhythmias, or abnormal heart rhythms, which can lead to sudden cardiac death. Additionally, omega-3 fatty acids have been shown to lower blood pressure and improve arterial function, thereby reducing the risk of stroke and heart attack.

For individuals looking to increase their intake of omega-3 fatty acids, incorporating fatty fish into their diet a few times per week is an excellent strategy. Grilling or baking fish like salmon, trout, or herring can provide a delicious and heart-healthy source of EPA and DHA. For those who prefer plant-based sources, adding flaxseeds or chia seeds to smoothies, oatmeal, or yogurt can boost the intake of ALA.

For individuals who may not consume enough omega-3 fatty

acids through dietary sources, supplementation can be a viable option. Fish oil supplements are widely available and can provide concentrated doses of EPA and DHA. It's important to consult with a healthcare provider before starting any new supplement regimen to ensure it is safe and appropriate for individual health needs.

In addition to fish and plant-based sources, other foods fortified with omega-3 fatty acids, such as certain brands of eggs and dairy products, can offer an alternative way to increase intake. These fortified foods provide an accessible option for individuals who may not have regular access to fresh fish or nuts.

In conclusion, increasing the intake of omega-3 fatty acids is a valuable strategy for promoting heart health. Whether through dietary sources, fortified foods, or supplements, incorporating these essential fatty acids into one's routine can contribute to a healthy heart and overall well-being. By embracing diverse sources of omega-3 fatty acids, individuals can take proactive steps to support their cardiovascular health and reduce the risk of heart disease.

2.3. Reducing Sodium Intake

Sodium, a mineral commonly found in salt, is an essential nutrient for the body. However, excessive consumption of sodium can have detrimental effects on heart health. High levels of sodium intake are associated with increased blood pressure, which can lead to a higher risk of heart disease, stroke, and other cardiovascular problems. Therefore, it is crucial to be mindful of sodium intake and take proactive steps to reduce it for a healthier heart.

One of the most significant sources of sodium in the diet is processed and packaged foods. Items such as canned soups, pre-packaged snacks, frozen meals, and condiments often contain high levels of sodium as a preservative and flavor enhancer. By choosing fresh, whole foods and preparing meals at home, individuals can have better control over their sodium intake. Incorporating a variety of herbs, spices, and citrus juices can add flavor to dishes without the need for excessive salt.

Another important consideration is reading food labels carefully. Many products that appear to be healthy may still contain high levels of sodium. Checking the sodium content per serving and being mindful of portion sizes can help individuals make informed choices about the foods they consume.

In addition to avoiding processed foods and monitoring labels, individuals can also reduce sodium intake by limiting the use of table salt and high-sodium condiments. Experimenting with alternative seasonings such as garlic, onion, black pepper, and lemon juice can enhance the taste of meals without relying solely on salt.

Restaurant meals are another

potential source of hidden sodium. Dishes prepared outside the home often contain unexpectedly high levels of salt. Asking for dressings and sauces on the side, opting for grilled or steamed dishes, and inquiring about the sodium content of menu items can all help in making more heart-healthy choices when dining out.

It's also important to note that not all salts are created equal. While reducing the overall intake of sodium is recommended, choosing high-quality, mineral-rich salts such as Himalayan pink salt or sea salt in moderation can provide additional nutrients and flavor compared to refined table salt.

In summary, reducing sodium intake is a vital step towards maintaining a healthy heart. By being mindful of food choices, cooking at home, reading labels, and being cautious of hidden sources of sodium, individuals can take proactive measures to support their cardiovascular well-being.

Embracing a varied and flavorful diet without relying heavily on salt can not only benefit heart health but also contribute to overall wellness. With dedication and conscious effort, individuals can significantly reduce their sodium intake and pave the way for a healthier heart and a healthier life.

2.4. Incorporating More Fruits and Vegetables

A diet rich in fruits and vegetables is widely recognized as beneficial for heart health. These nutrient-dense foods are packed with essential vitamins, minerals, fiber, and antioxidants that contribute to overall well-being and support cardiovascular health. By incorporating a variety of colorful fruits and vegetables into one's daily meals, individuals can take proactive steps towards maintaining a healthy heart and reducing the risk of heart disease.

The benefits of fruits and vegetables for heart health are multifaceted. Firstly, high consumption of these plant-based foods has been associated with lower blood pressure. The potassium content in fruits such as bananas, oranges, and kiwi, as well as in vegetables like sweet potatoes, spinach, and tomatoes, plays a key role in regulating blood pressure levels. Additionally, the high fiber content in fruits and vegetables can help lower cholesterol levels, reduce the risk of developing plaque in the arteries, and aid in weight management, all of which are crucial factors in maintaining heart health.

Furthermore, fruits and vegetables are rich in an array of powerful antioxidants, such as vitamin C, vitamin E, and various phytochemicals, which help protect against oxidative stress and inflammation in the body. These compounds have been shown to support overall cardiovascular function and reduce the risk of heart disease. For example, berries are known for their high antioxidant content, particularly anthocyanins, which have been linked to improved heart health and reduced risk of cardiovascular disease.

In addition to their nutritional benefits, fruits and vegetables can be incredibly versatile and delicious, making it easier to incorporate them into one's diet. From fresh salads and smoothies to roasted vegetables and fruit-based desserts, there are countless ways to enjoy these natural foods and reap their heart-healthy benefits. Embracing a wide variety of fruits and vegetables can also introduce a spectrum of flavors and textures to meals, making eating a more enjoyable and satisfying experience.

When striving to incorporate more fruits and vegetables into one's diet, it's important to prioritize variety and diversity. Different fruits and vegetables offer distinct nutritional profiles, so consuming an assortment of colors and types ensures that the body receives a broad spectrum of essential nutrients. For example, dark leafy greens like kale and spinach provide ample amounts of vitamin K and folate, while orange-colored produce like carrots and pumpkin are rich sources of beta-carotene and vitamin A. By regularly consuming a wide range of fruits and vegetables, individuals can optimize their intake of essential nutrients that contribute to heart health.

To make it easier to increase fruit and vegetable consumption, individuals can consider meal planning and preparation as a way to ensure that these foods are readily available and incorporated into daily meals. This may involve setting aside time each week to wash, chop, and store a variety of fruits and vegetables, making them easily accessible for snacking and cooking. Additionally, exploring local farmers' markets and grocery stores can provide opportunities to discover fresh, seasonal produce and inspire new culinary creations.

In conclusion, incorporating more

fruits and vegetables into one's diet is a powerful and enjoyable way to support heart health. By providing essential nutrients, fiber, antioxidants, and flavor, these natural foods play a crucial role in promoting overall cardiovascular well-being. With a mindful approach to dietary choices and a commitment to diversifying fruit and vegetable consumption, individuals can take proactive steps towards nurturing a healthy heart and enjoying the numerous benefits of a plant-rich diet.

2.5. Choosing Whole Grains over Refined Grains

Choosing Whole Grains over Refined Grains for a Healthy Heart Diet

One of the most effective ways to maintain a healthy heart is through a balanced and nutritious diet. While all nutrients play a vital role, carbohydrates, especially grains, have a significant impact on heart health. However, not all grains are created equal. Whole grains offer superior health benefits compared to refined grains and should be the primary choice for individuals aiming to maintain a healthy heart.

Whole grains are grains that contain all parts of the kernel – the bran, germ, and endosperm. This means they retain vital nutrients such as fiber, vitamins, minerals, and antioxidants. Refined grains, on the other hand, undergo processing that removes the bran and germ, leaving only the endosperm. This process eliminates a significant amount of nutrients, resulting in a less nutritious grain.

To understand why whole grains should be favored over refined grains for a healthy heart diet, it is essential to examine their impact on heart health. Whole grains are an excellent source of dietary fiber, which plays a crucial role in maintaining a healthy cardiovascular system. Fiber helps lower cholesterol levels by preventing its reabsorption in the bloodstream, thus reducing the risk of heart disease. Additionally, the fiber in whole grains promotes satiety and weight management, which further contributes to a healthy heart.

Refined grains, on the other hand, contain little to no dietary fiber after processing, leaving them nutritionally depleted. Consuming these grains regularly can contribute to higher cholesterol levels, obesity, and increased risk of heart disease. The refined nature of these grains significantly impacts blood sugar levels, leading to rapid spikes and crashes, which may increase the risk of developing diabetes – a condition closely linked to heart disease.

When incorporating whole grains into a healthy heart diet, individuals should aim to consume a variety of options. Whole wheat, oatmeal, brown rice, barley, quinoa, and whole grain pasta are excellent choices that provide an array of nutrients while maintaining heart health. These grains can be consumed in various forms, including bread, cereals, or as whole grains in meals, allowing for flexibility in meal planning.

It is important to note that some products labeled as "whole grain" may still contain refined grains. Reading product labels carefully and opting for ingredients like whole wheat flour or whole oats ensures the consumption of genuinely whole grain products. Incorporating these choices into a well-balanced diet, alongside other heart-healthy foods, such as fruits, vegetables, lean proteins, and healthy fats, will enhance cardiovascular health.

In conclusion, choosing whole grains

over refined grains is essential for maintaining a healthy heart diet. Whole grains are rich in fiber and retain valuable nutrients, while refined grains lack essential components, making them less nutritious. By prioritizing whole grains such as whole wheat, oatmeal, and brown rice, individuals can promote heart health, lower cholesterol levels, and reduce the risk of heart disease. Remember, making a conscious choice to include whole grains in daily meals is a step towards a healthier heart and overall well-being.

2.6. Including Lean Proteins in Your Diet

Protein is an essential macronutrient that plays a crucial role in maintaining your overall health. Incorporating lean proteins into your diet is a great way to ensure your body gets the amino acids it needs while avoiding unnecessary fats and calories. In this chapter, we will explore the importance of lean proteins, their benefits, and how to incorporate them into your daily meals.

Understanding Lean Proteins:

Lean proteins are rich in essential amino acids and low in unhealthy fats. They are vital for muscle growth and repair, regulating hormones, maintaining a healthy weight, and supporting a strong immune system. Unlike fatty meats or processed proteins, lean proteins offer numerous health benefits without the risk of increased cholesterol levels or weight gain.

Benefits of Lean Proteins:

1. Weight Management: Lean proteins are highly satiating, meaning they keep you feeling full for longer periods. By incorporating lean proteins into your diet, you reduce hunger pangs and prevent unnecessary snacking. This leads to better weight management and can help in achieving weight loss goals.

2. Muscle Building: If you're engaging in regular exercise, consuming lean proteins assists in muscle repair and growth. After a workout, protein helps repair the

micro-damage that occurs in your muscles, contributing to their development and overall strength.

3. Blood Sugar Regulation: Compared to carbohydrates, proteins have a minimal effect on blood sugar levels. When consumed alongside carbohydrates, lean proteins can aid in stabilizing your blood glucose levels, reducing the risk of diabetes and promoting sustained energy throughout the day.

4. Positive Impact on Heart Health:

Lean proteins, such as chicken breast, turkey, fish, beans, and legumes, have been associated with improved heart health. They contain essential nutrients like omega-3 fatty acids and unsaturated fats, which can reduce inflammation and contribute to maintaining healthy blood pressure and cholesterol levels.

Incorporating Lean Proteins into Your Diet:

1. Choose Lean Protein Sources: Opt for lean animal proteins like skinless

chicken or turkey breast, fish, and low-fat dairy products. Furthermore, plant-based sources like tofu, tempeh, legumes, and soy products are excellent alternatives for vegans and vegetarians.

2. Balanced Meal Planning: Aim to include lean proteins in each of your main meals. For instance, whole grains paired with chicken breast and roasted vegetables or a salad with grilled fish can make for a nutritious and well-rounded meal.

3. Snack Smart: If you're feeling

hungry between meals, consider protein-rich snacks to keep you satiated. Options can include Greek yogurt, cottage cheese, hard-boiled eggs, a handful of nuts, or a protein shake.

4. Prioritize Variety: Don't limit your protein sources to just one or two options. Explore different lean protein sources to maintain a healthy and diverse diet. This allows you to benefit from a wide range of nutrients while preventing taste fatigue.

5. Cook with Healthy Methods: Opt for cooking methods that preserve the nutritional value of lean proteins. Grilling, baking, broiling, or steaming are great alternatives to frying, as they promote healthier meals without added fats.

Incorporating lean proteins into your diet is a wise choice for maintaining optimal health. These protein sources offer several benefits, ranging from weight management to improved heart health. By selecting lean proteins, planning balanced meals, and incorporating protein-rich snacks, you can easily ensure your body receives the right amount of protein for its daily needs. Remember to prioritize variety and cook with healthy methods to maximize the nutritional benefits.

2.7. Monitoring and Limiting Added Sugars

Monitoring and limiting added sugars is an essential aspect of maintaining a healthy heart diet. Excessive consumption of added sugars has been linked to various health issues, including heart disease, obesity, and type 2 diabetes. In this chapter, we will explore the importance of monitoring and limiting added sugars in a healthy heart diet and provide practical strategies to achieve this goal.

Understanding Added Sugars:

Before we delve into monitoring and limiting added sugars, it is vital to understand what added sugars are. Added sugars refer to the sugars and syrups that are added to foods and beverages during their processing or preparation. These sugars are not naturally present in the food and provide empty calories without any nutritional value.

The Negative Effects of Added Sugars on the Heart:

Excessive consumption of added sugars can have severe repercussions on heart health. Research has shown a direct correlation between high sugar intake and an increased risk of developing heart disease. Added sugars lead to chronic inflammation, elevated blood pressure, increased triglyceride levels, and weight gain. These factors contribute to the development of cardiovascular problems such as atherosclerosis, heart attacks, and strokes. Therefore, it is crucial to monitor and limit added sugar intake to maintain a healthy heart.

Monitoring Added Sugars:

To effectively monitor added sugar intake, it is important to be aware of hidden sources of sugar. Many packaged foods, such as cereals, snack bars, condiments, and beverages, contain high amounts of added sugars. Take the time to read food labels and identify ingredients such as sucrose, high fructose corn syrup, dextrose, and other names for added sugars. Be cautious of foods marketed as "low fat" or "diet" alternatives, as they often compensate for the lack of taste by adding extra sugar.

Limiting Added Sugars:

Reducing added sugar consumption may seem challenging, but with the right approach and mindset, it is achievable. Here are some strategies to limit added sugars in a healthy heart diet:

1. Opt for Whole Foods: Choose whole, unprocessed foods whenever possible. Fruits, vegetables, lean proteins, and whole grains provide essential nutrients and are naturally low in added sugars.

2. Sweeten Naturally: Instead of reaching for sugary drinks or adding

sugar to foods, try natural sweeteners like stevia, honey, or maple syrup in moderation. Remember that even natural sweeteners should be consumed in limited quantities as they still contain sugar.

3. Cook at Home: Preparing meals at home allows you to control the ingredients and avoid hidden sugars. Choose homemade sauces, dressings, and marinades over store-bought options, which often contain added sugars.

4. Read Food Labels: Familiarize yourself with reading food labels and make it a habit to check the sugar content of packaged foods. Look for products with no added sugars or those that contain minimal amounts.

5. Be Mindful of Beverages: Beverages, such as soda, fruit juices, and flavored coffees, are often packed with added sugars. Opt for water, unsweetened tea, or infused water to quench your thirst without the added sugar.

6. Practice Moderation: It's important to remember that moderation is key. While it is crucial to limit added sugars, completely eliminating them from your diet may not be practical or necessary. Allow yourself occasional treats, but keep them as an occasional indulgence rather than a regular part of your diet.

Monitoring and limiting added sugars are essential steps in maintaining a healthy heart diet. By being aware of hidden sources of added sugars, making conscious food choices, and practicing moderation, you can significantly reduce your intake of added sugars and protect your heart health. Stay mindful of the sugar content in the foods you consume and focus on nourishing your body with whole, nutritious foods to maintain a healthy heart and overall well-being.

Chapter 3

Planning Your Heart Healthy Meals

3.1. Creating Balanced and Nutritious Meals

Eating a balanced and nutritious diet is crucial for maintaining a healthy heart. Although it may seem overwhelming at first, understanding the key components of a heart-healthy meal can greatly contribute to your overall well-being. In this chapter, we will explore various strategies to create meals that are not only delicious but also promote optimal heart health.

1. The Foundation of a Heart-Healthy Meal:

The first step in creating balanced and nutritious meals is establishing a solid foundation. This entails incorporating whole foods such as fruits, vegetables, whole grains, lean proteins, and healthy fats into your diet. These foods provide essential nutrients, fiber, and antioxidants that can help reduce the risk of heart disease.

2. The Power of Plant-Based Foods:

Plant-based foods should take center stage in your heart-healthy meals. Fruits and vegetables not only provide important vitamins, minerals, and fiber but are also low in calories and high in antioxidants. Aim to incorporate a variety of colorful produce into each meal, including leafy greens, berries, citrus fruits, cruciferous vegetables, and sweet potatoes.

3. Embracing Whole Grains:

Swap refined grains for whole grains

to maximize the nutritional value of your meals. Whole grains, such as quinoa, brown rice, whole wheat bread, and oats, are rich in fiber and can help lower LDL (bad) cholesterol levels. Experiment with different whole grains to add diversity and flavor to your meals.

4. Opting for Lean Proteins:

Protein is an essential building block for our bodies, but it's important to choose lean sources. Opt for skinless poultry, fish like salmon or mackerel, legumes, and tofu. These options are low in saturated fats and cholesterol, making them heart-healthy choices. Additionally, fish contains omega-3 fatty acids, which have been linked to a reduced risk of heart disease.

5. The Role of Healthy Fats:

Contrary to popular belief, not all fats are created equal. Healthy fats, such as those found in avocados, nuts, seeds, and olive oil, are beneficial for heart health. These fats help lower LDL cholesterol levels while raising HDL (good) cholesterol levels. Incorporating these fats in moderation can boost the nutritional profile of your meals.

6. Portion Control and Mindful Eating:

Even with a well-balanced meal, portion control plays a vital role in maintaining heart health. Moderation is key when it comes to portion sizes, especially with calorie-dense foods. Practice mindful eating by slowing down, savoring each bite, and being aware of your body's satiety cues. This will help prevent overeating and promote healthier eating habits.

7. Combining Nutrients for Maximum Benefit:

To create optimal heart-healthy meals, aim for a combination of nutrients in each dish. For example, pair lean protein with whole grain carbohydrates and a generous serving of vegetables. This balanced combination will provide sustained energy while keeping you full and satisfied.

Creating balanced and nutritious

meals for heart health is a journey that requires patience, experimentation, and a willingness to prioritize your well-being. By incorporating whole foods, focusing on plants, embracing whole grains, choosing lean proteins, including healthy fats, practicing portion control, and combining nutrients effectively, you'll be on your way to a healthier heart and a happier, more vibrant life. Remember, small changes in your eating habits can lead to significant improvements in your overall cardiovascular health.

3.2. Portion Control and Moderation

When it comes to maintaining a heart-healthy diet, the importance of portion control and moderation cannot be overstated. While it is essential to choose the right foods for your heart, it is equally important to consume them in appropriate amounts. In this chapter, we will explore the principles of portion control and moderation, and how they can contribute to a long and healthy life.

Understanding Portion Control:

Portion control refers to the practice of eating an appropriate amount of food to meet your body's nutritional needs without overindulging. In today's society, portion sizes have grown significantly, contributing to the rise of obesity and various heart diseases. It's vital to retrain ourselves on what constitutes a proper serving size to maintain a healthy weight and support cardiovascular health.

One simple way to visualize portion

sizes is to use our own hands as a guide. For instance, a serving of protein, such as chicken or fish, should be approximately the size of our palm. A serving of carbohydrates, like rice or pasta, should be about the size of our closed fist. By using this practical approach, we can avoid overeating and ensure appropriate portion sizes.

The Role of Moderation:

While portion control is essential, it is also crucial to practice moderation when it comes to less healthy food choices. No diet should prohibit all indulgences, as this can lead to feelings of deprivation and ultimately, failure. Moderation allows us to enjoy occasional treats while still maintaining a heart-healthy lifestyle.

Moderation means enjoying foods that may not be as beneficial to our cardiovascular health in smaller quantities and less frequently. For example, it is reasonable to savor a small piece of dark chocolate or have a slice of cake on special occasions. By managing our indulgences in this way, we can strike a balance between enjoying life's pleasures and maintaining our cardiovascular well-being.

Tips for Putting Portion Control and Moderation into Practice:

1. Read food labels: Pay attention to the suggested serving sizes listed on food packaging. This will help you understand what a proper portion looks like and prevent overeating.

2. Use smaller plates: Eating off smaller plates tricks our minds into

thinking we are consuming more food, helping us feel satisfied with smaller portions.

3. Listen to your body: Pay attention to your body's hunger and fullness cues. Eat until you are comfortably full, but not overstuffed.

4. Slow down and savor: Eating slowly and mindfully can help you enjoy your food more while also allowing your brain to register when you've had enough.

5. Plan indulgences: Allocate specific occasions or commitments for

enjoying your favorite treats. This will help you control portion sizes and prevent overindulgence.

Note: Portion control and moderation are pivotal aspects of maintaining a heart-healthy diet. By understanding appropriate portion sizes, practicing moderation in our eating habits, and implementing practical strategies, we can successfully navigate our way to improved cardiovascular health. So, let us embrace moderation, listen to our bodies, and savor every bite as we embark on this journey towards a heart-healthy lifestyle.

3.3. Meal Prepping for Heart Health

In today's fast-paced world, it's easy to succumb to unhealthy eating habits and convenience foods that are detrimental to our heart health. However, with a little planning and dedication, we can take control of our diets and improve our cardiovascular well-being. Enter meal prepping! In this chapter, we'll explore the art of meal prepping for heart health, providing you with practical tips, delicious recipes, and expert advice to keep your heart happy and healthy.

Part 1: The Importance of Meal Prepping for Heart Health

1.1 Understanding the Connection between Diet and Heart Health: We delve into the relationship between the food we eat and our cardiovascular system, highlighting the dietary factors that can promote heart disease or protect against it.

1.2 Benefits of Meal Prepping for Heart Health: Exploring the numerous advantages of meal prepping, such as better portion control, reduced reliance on processed foods, cost-effectiveness, and time-saving benefits.

Part 2: Essential Components of a Heart-Healthy Meal Plan

2.1 Incorporating Whole Foods: Learn about the importance of including whole grains, lean proteins, fruits, vegetables, and healthy fats in your meal prepping routine to support heart health.

2.2 Balancing Macronutrients:

Understanding how to balance carbohydrates, proteins, and fats in your meals, ensuring a well-rounded approach to heart-healthy nutrition.

2.3 Sodium and Sugar Reduction: Practical strategies for minimizing sodium and added sugars in your diet, explaining their detrimental effects on cardiovascular health and suggesting healthier alternatives.

Part 3: Meal Prep Tips and Techniques

3.1 Start with a Plan: A step-by-step guide to creating a heart-healthy meal plan, including setting goals, identifying recipes, and making a grocery list.

3.2 Efficient Meal Prepping: Proven techniques to streamline the meal prepping process, such as batch cooking, prepping ingredients in advance, and utilizing kitchen tools effectively.

3.3 Storage and Safety: Tips for proper food storage, labeling, and handling to ensure both freshness and food safety.

Part 4: Delicious Heart-Healthy Meal

Prep Recipes

4.1 Breakfast on-the-go: Quick and nutritious breakfast options for busy mornings, including make-ahead smoothie packs, overnight oats, and vegetable frittatas.

4.2 Satisfying Lunches: Vibrant and filling salad jars, wrap sandwiches, and grain-based Buddha bowls that are packed with heart-healthy ingredients.

4.3 Nourishing Dinners: Flavorful and wholesome dinner recipes, such as baked salmon with roasted vegetables, vegetarian chili, and quinoa-stuffed bell peppers.

4.4 Guilt-Free Snacks: Snack ideas that satisfy cravings without compromising heart health, including homemade granola bars, roasted chickpeas, and fruit skewers.

Finally, meal prepping for heart health is a game-changer, enabling you to take charge of your diet and ultimately protect your cardiovascular system. By understanding the link between nutrition and heart health, incorporating essential components into your meals, and mastering the art of meal prepping, you can enjoy delicious, heart-healthy meals every day. So, put on your apron, grab your containers, and embark on a journey towards a healthier heart, one prepped meal at a time.

Chapter 4.

Staying Hydrated and Limiting Alcohol Consumption

In the pursuit of a healthy heart, there are various aspects to consider, from exercise and diet to stress management and sleep patterns. However, one often overlooked factor that plays a significant role in maintaining a healthy heart is proper hydration and limiting alcohol consumption. In this chapter, we will delve into the importance of staying hydrated, explore its benefits for cardiovascular health, and discuss the detrimental effects of excessive alcohol intake. By understanding the relationship between hydration, alcohol consumption, and heart health, you can make informed choices to optimize your well-being.

The Essence of Hydration:

Water is the essence of life, and it is vital for our bodies to function efficiently. Our hearts, like all other organs, depend on a steady supply of water to perform optimally. The cardiovascular system relies on adequate hydration to maintain proper blood volume and pressure, ensuring efficient blood circulation throughout the body. Dehydration, on the other hand, can lead to thickening of the blood, increased strain on the heart, and heightened risk of cardiac complications.

Benefits of Staying Hydrated:

1. Blood pressure regulation: Drinking enough water helps to maintain normal blood pressure levels, reducing the strain on your

heart and decreasing the risk of cardiovascular diseases.

2. Improved circulation: When the body is adequately hydrated, blood flows smoothly, delivering oxygen and essential nutrients to the heart and other organs. Good blood circulation also helps the heart in efficiently removing waste products from the body, enhancing overall cardiovascular health.

3. Enhanced exercise performance: Proper hydration helps your muscles work more efficiently during

physical activity. By staying hydrated, you can exercise for longer durations while experiencing less fatigue and preventing unnecessary stress on your heart.

4. Optimal heart rhythm: Water plays a crucial role in maintaining the electrolyte balance necessary for proper heart rhythm. Adequate hydration can help prevent arrhythmias and other irregularities.

5. Enhanced kidney function: The kidneys, responsible for filtering waste products from the

bloodstream, function optimally when the body is well-hydrated. This indirectly aids heart health by promoting overall detoxification and waste removal.

The Pitfalls of Alcohol Consumption:

While moderate alcohol consumption has been associated with potential cardiovascular benefits, excessive or chronic alcohol intake can be detrimental to heart health. Here are some reasons why alcohol should be consumed in moderation:

1. Increased blood pressure: Regular heavy drinking can cause high blood pressure, leading to an increased risk of heart disease, stroke, and heart failure.

2. Weakened heart muscles: Alcohol damages heart muscle cells, leading to a condition called alcoholic cardiomyopathy. This weakens the heart's ability to pump blood effectively and can eventually result in heart failure.

3. Irregular heart rhythm: Alcohol consumption can cause

disturbances in heart rhythm, known as arrhythmias. These irregular heartbeats can be dangerous and may increase the risk of stroke or cardiac arrest.

4. Weight gain and increased triglyceride levels: Alcoholic beverages are often high in calories and can contribute to weight gain when consumed in excess. This weight gain, combined with increased triglyceride levels associated with alcohol consumption, can further strain the

cardiovascular system.

Practical Tips for Staying Hydrated and Limiting Alcohol Consumption:

1. Drink water frequently throughout the day, aiming for at least eight glasses (64 ounces) to ensure adequate hydration.

2. Substitute alcoholic beverages with healthier alternatives such as flavored water, herbal tea, or sparkling water infused with fruits to satisfy your taste buds while reducing alcohol intake.

3. Be vigilant of your alcohol consumption and set limits. Moderation is key – for men, this means up to two standard drinks per day, while women should consume no more than one.

4. If consuming alcohol, hydrate alongside by drinking water before, during, and after to counteract its dehydrating effects.

5. Engage in mindful drinking practices, considering alcohol-free days and choosing quality over quantity.

Note: Staying hydrated and limiting alcohol consumption are crucial for maintaining a healthy heart. By understanding the benefits of hydration and the pitfalls of excessive alcohol intake, you can make informed decisions that promote cardiovascular well-being. So, raise your glass of water and toast to a heart that beats strong and vibrantly – a testament to your commitment to staying hydrated and making responsible choices.

Chapter 5.

Reducing Stress and Incorporating Physical Activity

In today's fast-paced and demanding world, stress has become an integral part of our lives. However, the toll it takes on our overall health, especially our heart health, cannot be overlooked. Chronic stress has been linked to an increased risk of cardiovascular diseases and can lead to the development of more severe conditions, such as hypertension and heart attacks. Therefore, it is crucial to find effective strategies to reduce stress and incorporate physical activity into our daily routines for the benefit of our hearts.

The Vicious Cycle of Stress and Heart Health:

Stress triggers the release of stress hormones, such as cortisol and adrenaline, which prepare our bodies for the fight or flight response. While this response is essential in emergency situations, experiencing it chronically can have detrimental effects on our cardiovascular system. The increased heart rate, elevated blood pressure, and constricted blood vessels associated with stress can strain the heart and potentially lead to long-term damage.

Recognizing and Managing Stress:

Before we can effectively reduce stress, it is important to recognize its presence in our lives. Often, stress becomes so normalized that we fail to acknowledge its impact on our health. In this chapter, we will explore various stress management techniques, such as meditation, deep breathing exercises, and engaging in hobbies or activities that bring us joy. By incorporating these practices into our daily routines, we can develop healthier coping mechanisms that promote heart health.

Physical Activity as a Stress Reliever:

Engaging in regular physical activity is not only essential for heart health but also highly effective in reducing stress levels. Exercise stimulates the production of endorphins—natural mood-enhancers—which can combat stress and improve our overall well-being. In this chapter, we will delve into different forms of exercise, including cardiovascular activities like running or swimming, strength training, and mind-body exercises such as yoga and tai chi. We will explore how each type of activity can contribute to stress reduction and heart health.

Creating Sustainable Active Habits:

Incorporating physical activity into our daily lives can be challenging, especially when we are already stressed and pressed for time. However, it is crucial to prioritize our heart health and find ways to make exercise a natural part of our routines. This chapter will provide practical tips and strategies for incorporating physical activity into our busy schedules. We will discuss simple changes such as taking the stairs instead of the elevator, scheduling regular workout sessions, and finding enjoyable physical activities that resonate with our interests and preferences.

The Role of Social Support:

When it comes to reducing stress and making lifestyle changes for heart health, social support plays a significant role. Having a supportive network of friends, family, or joining exercise groups can provide the motivation and accountability necessary for maintaining a physically active lifestyle. We will explore the benefits of social support, ways to build a support system, and how it can positively impact our overall well-being.

Finally, reducing stress and incorporating physical activity into our daily lives are vital steps in protecting our heart health. By consciously managing our stress levels through stress reduction techniques and engaging in regular exercise, we can cultivate a healthier and happier lifestyle. The benefits extend beyond the cardiovascular system, improving our overall well-being and quality of life. Through the implementation of the strategies discussed in this chapter, we can reduce stress, boost our heart health, and create sustainable habits that promote lifelong well-being.

Chapter 6.

Healthy Cooking Techniques for Heart Health

In today's fast-paced world, many of us prioritize convenience over health when it comes to our meals. However, with a growing concern for cardiovascular health, it is essential to adopt cooking techniques that not only preserve the nutritional value of our foods but also promote heart health. In this chapter, we will explore some exciting and innovative cooking techniques that will help you maintain a happy and healthy heart.

1. Grilling: A Flavorful, Heart-Healthy Option

Grilling is a fantastic technique that imparts a smoky flavor to your foods without excessive use of added fats. When grilling, choose lean proteins such as skinless chicken, fish, or tofu, which are high in omega-3 fatty acids known to reduce the risk of heart disease. To enhance the flavors, marinate your proteins with a mixture of herbs, spices, and citrus juices, instead of relying on heavy sauces and dressings which can be high in sodium and unhealthy fats. Grilled vegetables like peppers, zucchini, and eggplants are also rich in fiber and antioxidants, making them excellent choices for heart health.

2. Steaming: Retaining Nutrients and Flavor

Steaming is an ideal cooking technique for heart-healthy meals, as it requires minimal fat and preserves the nutritional value of ingredients. By steaming vegetables, you ensure that they retain their natural vitamins and minerals, like potassium and magnesium, which are essential for heart health. Additionally, steaming fish or whole grains like quinoa or brown rice can result in a delicious and heart-friendly meal. Experiment with different herbs and spices to add flavor, and consider using vegetable or chicken broth in place of plain water for an added depth of taste.

3. Stir-Frying: Quick and Nourishing

Stir-frying is a versatile technique that allows you to cook heart-healthy meals within a matter of minutes. By using minimal oil and high heat, you can quickly cook a variety of colorful vegetables while retaining their nutritional value. Consider using heart-healthy oils like olive oil or avocado oil, which contain monounsaturated fats known for reducing cholesterol levels. To add protein to your stir-fries, opt for lean meats like chicken or turkey, or try tofu or tempeh for a plant-based option. Enhance the flavors by using ginger, garlic, and low-sodium soy sauce, and serve your stir-fries over a bed of nutrient-rich whole grains.

4. Baking: A Heart-Friendly Alternative

Baking is a fantastic heart-healthy cooking technique that allows you to eliminate excessive fat while retaining flavors and textures. For healthier baked goods, swap out oil or butter for healthier alternatives like applesauce, mashed bananas, or Greek yogurt. Similarly, replace refined flours with whole-wheat or nut flours, which offer higher amounts of fiber and essential nutrients. Baking heart-healthy desserts, such as fruit crisps with oatmeal as a topping or dark chocolate-dipped strawberries, can help satisfy sweet cravings while protecting your cardiovascular health.

Modern cooking techniques have evolved to prioritize convenience and taste, often at the expense of our heart health. However, by adopting innovative techniques such as grilling, steaming, stir-frying, and baking, we can create delicious and heart-healthy meals without sacrificing flavor. So, unleash your culinary creativity and embark on a journey towards a healthier heart, one dish at a time. Your taste buds and cardiovascular system will thank you for it!

Chapter 7.

Sample Meal Plans and Recipes for a Heart Healthy Diet

Eating a heart-healthy diet is crucial for maintaining optimal heart health and reducing the risk of cardiovascular diseases. A well-balanced meal plan with nutrient-dense foods can help lower cholesterol levels, reduce blood pressure, and promote overall cardiovascular wellness. In this chapter, we will explore sample meal plans and provide delicious and nutritious recipes to make your heart-healthy journey enjoyable and sustainable.

Sample Meal Plan 1: Mediterranean-inspired Delights

The Mediterranean diet is lauded for its heart-healthy benefits. This meal plan incorporates its principles and flavors.

Breakfast:

- Greek yogurt parfait with fresh fruits and granola: Layer Greek yogurt, berries, sliced banana, and whole-grain granola for a satisfying and protein-packed start to your day.

- Herbal tea or green tea for added antioxidants.

Lunch:

- Mediterranean hummus and roasted vegetable wrap: Spread hummus onto a whole-grain tortilla and fill it with roasted peppers, eggplant, zucchini, and spinach. Roll it up for a tasty and portable lunch.

- Mixed green salad with feta cheese and a drizzle of olive oil and lemon juice.

Snack:

- Raw almonds and dried apricots: A handful of nutrient-dense almonds and dried fruits provide a satisfying snack that will keep you energized and full until your next meal.

Dinner:

- Grilled salmon with lemon and dill: Marinate salmon fillets in lemon juice, garlic, and fresh dill, then grill until tender and flaky. Serve with steamed asparagus and quinoa for a complete heart-healthy meal.

- Roasted sweet potatoes with a sprinkle of cinnamon and a side salad of mixed greens.

Dessert:

- Fresh fruit salad with a dollop of Greek yogurt: Enjoy a mix of colorful fruits such as berries, melons, and citrus fruits for a refreshing and nutritious dessert.

Sample Meal Plan 2: Plant-Based Powerhouse

A plant-based diet can significantly

improve heart health, as it is low in saturated fats and high in fiber and antioxidants. This meal plan illustrates how delicious and satisfying plant-based eating can be.

Breakfast:

- Overnight chia seed pudding: Mix chia seeds with your choice of plant-based milk, a touch of honey or maple syrup, and a splash of vanilla extract. Let it sit overnight, and in the morning, top with fresh fruit, nuts, and seeds.

- Herbal tea or freshly squeezed juice

for a vibrant start.

Lunch:

- Chickpea and vegetable curry: Sauté onions, garlic, and ginger in a pot. Add diced vegetables like bell peppers, carrots, and zucchini, along with canned chickpeas. Season with curry powder, turmeric, and coconut milk. Simmer until vegetables are tender. Serve over brown rice or quinoa.

- Steamed broccoli or a side salad with a tangy vinaigrette.

Snack:

- Sliced cucumber and hummus: Dip cucumber slices into homemade or store-bought hummus for a refreshing and heart-healthy snack.

Dinner:

- Lentil and vegetable stir-fry: Sauté onions, bell peppers, snap peas, and mushrooms. Add cooked lentils and season with soy sauce, garlic, and ginger. Serve over whole-wheat noodles or brown rice.

- Roasted Brussels sprouts with a

drizzle of balsamic glaze.

Dessert:

- Baked cinnamon apple slices: Core and slice apples, then toss with a sprinkle of cinnamon and bake until tender. Enjoy with a scoop of dairy-free vanilla ice cream or a dollop of coconut whipped cream.

These sample meal plans and recipes demonstrate that a heart-healthy diet doesn't have to be boring or restrictive. By incorporating nutrient-dense foods, lean proteins, and plenty of fruits and vegetables, you can create delicious and satisfying meals that promote heart health and overall wellness. Remember to customize these plans based on your dietary preferences and consult with a healthcare professional for personalized advice. Enjoy exploring new flavors and embracing a heart-healthy lifestyle.

Chapter 8.

Special Considerations for Individuals with Specific Heart Conditions

Proper nutrition plays a crucial role in maintaining heart health and managing specific heart conditions. While a balanced diet is important for everyone, individuals with certain heart conditions need to pay special attention to their meal choices. In this chapter, we will explore the unique dietary considerations for individuals with specific heart conditions and provide practical tips for creating heart-healthy meals.

1. Hypertension: A Low-Sodium Lifestyle

High blood pressure, or hypertension, is a common heart condition that can greatly increase the risk of heart disease and stroke. One of the key dietary interventions for managing hypertension is reducing sodium intake. Excessive sodium consumption can cause fluid retention and contribute to elevated blood pressure levels.

To adhere to a low-sodium lifestyle, individuals with hypertension should focus on:

- Reading food labels: Pay close attention to the sodium content listed on packaged foods and choose low-sodium or sodium-free options whenever possible.

- Avoiding processed foods: Processed foods, such as canned soups, deli meats, and fast food, are often high in sodium. Opt for fresh, whole foods instead.

- Using herbs and spices: Enhance the flavor of meals with herbs, spices, and other salt-free seasonings to reduce the need for added sodium.

- Meal planning: Prepare homemade meals using fresh ingredients, allowing better control over sodium content.

2. High Cholesterol: The Battle Against Bad Fats

High cholesterol levels, specifically elevated levels of LDL (low-density lipoprotein) or "bad" cholesterol, are a significant risk factor for heart disease. To manage cholesterol levels, it is essential to limit the intake of saturated and trans fats, which can increase LDL cholesterol in the blood.

Consider the following dietary tips for individuals with high cholesterol:

- Choose healthy fats: Replace saturated and trans fats with healthier options, such as monounsaturated fats found in olive oil, avocados, and nuts, as well as polyunsaturated fats found in fatty fish, seeds, and vegetable oils.

- Incorporate plant sterols: Foods rich in plant sterols, such as whole grains, legumes, nuts, and seeds, can help lower LDL cholesterol levels.

- Increase fiber intake: Focus on consuming soluble fiber found in fruits, vegetables, whole grains, and legumes, as it can effectively decrease LDL cholesterol.

- Limit cholesterol-rich foods: Reduce the consumption of high-cholesterol foods like organ meats, shellfish, and fried foods.

3. Heart Failure: Managing Fluid Intake

Individuals with heart failure often need to adapt their diet to manage fluid retention and maintain healthy fluid balance. Heart failure can lead to excess fluid accumulation in the body, causing symptoms like swelling, shortness of breath, and fatigue. Regulating fluid intake is crucial to manage these symptoms effectively.

Consider the following dietary guidelines for individuals with heart failure:

- Moderating fluid intake: Consult with a healthcare professional to determine an appropriate fluid limit, typically around 1.5 to 2 liters per day, depending on individual needs.

- Monitoring electrolytes: Potassium and sodium levels play a significant role in fluid balance. Close attention should be paid to their intake to maintain proper electrolyte balance.

- Eating nutrient-dense, low-sodium

meals: Choose foods that provide necessary nutrients without excessive sodium, such as lean proteins, whole grains, vegetables, and fruits.

- Cooking methods: Opt for baking, grilling, or steaming instead of using sauces or gravies, which can be high in sodium.

4. Diabetes and Heart Health: Balancing Carbohydrates

Many individuals with heart conditions also have diabetes or prediabetes, requiring careful management of blood sugar levels alongside heart health. Balancing carbohydrate intake is crucial to regulate blood glucose levels while maintaining heart health.

Consider the following dietary strategies for individuals with diabetes and heart conditions:

- Choose whole grains: Opt for whole grains, such as quinoa, brown rice, and whole-wheat bread, over refined carbohydrates to improve both heart health and blood sugar control.

- Monitor portion sizes: Control carbohydrate portions to manage blood sugar levels effectively. Working with a registered dietitian can help create a personalized meal plan.

- Include lean proteins and healthy fats: Combining sources of lean proteins and healthy fats with carbohydrates can slow down digestion and prevent blood sugar spikes.

- Regular monitoring: Regularly

monitor blood glucose levels and make necessary adjustments to dietary choices and medication with the guidance of a healthcare professional.

Individuals with specific heart conditions need to be mindful of their dietary choices to manage their condition effectively. By following these special considerations and incorporating heart-healthy meals into their daily routine, individuals can promote heart health, manage their specific heart condition, and improve overall well-being. Remember, consulting with healthcare professionals, such as registered dietitians or cardiologists, is essential for maximum benefits and personalized dietary recommendations.

Chapter 9.

Tips for Dining Out and Traveling on a Heart Healthy Diet

Eating out and traveling can pose challenges when trying to maintain a heart healthy diet. With tempting menu options, large portion sizes, and limited healthy choices, it's easy to feel overwhelmed. However, with some simple strategies and a little planning, dining out and traveling can still be enjoyable while staying heart healthy. In this chapter, we will explore tips and tricks for navigating restaurants and unfamiliar environments to make heart-healthy choices.

1. Plan ahead:

Before heading out to a restaurant or embarking on a trip, it's crucial to do some research. Look for restaurants that offer heart-healthy options or that cater to specific dietary needs. Check online menus and reviews to get an idea of what dishes are available and how they are prepared. Consider packing healthy snacks for your travels, such as nuts, dried fruits, or granola bars, to avoid relying on unhealthy options during transit.

2. Be mindful of portion sizes:

Many restaurants serve portions that are much larger than recommended for a heart-healthy diet. To avoid overeating, try sharing a dish with a friend or ask for a half portion. Alternatively, divide the meal in half and save the rest for later. Avoid the temptation to finish everything on your plate just because it's served to you.

3. Choose wisely:

When dining out, select dishes that are prepared with heart-healthy ingredients and cooking methods. Look for items that are grilled, baked, broiled, steamed, or roasted instead of fried or sautéed. Opt for lean proteins like fish, chicken, or beans and plenty of fruits and vegetables. Avoid dishes that are high in sodium, saturated fats, or added sugars.

4. Customize your order:

Don't hesitate to ask for

modifications to suit your dietary needs. Ask for dressings and sauces to be served on the side, so you can control the amount you consume. Request that foods be cooked without added fats or salt. Feel confident in asking your server about the ingredients used or for any additional information regarding the dish's preparation.

5. Control temptations:

Resist the temptation to indulge in unhealthy options like breadbaskets or calorie-laden appetizers. Instead, ask for a side of fresh vegetables or a small salad to start. Choose water, unsweetened tea, or a glass of red wine over sugary sodas or cocktails. Savor a small portion of a healthy dessert, or consider sharing one with others at your table.

6. Be prepared while traveling:

When traveling, it's essential to plan for potential dietary challenges. Pack heart-healthy snacks for the journey, as well as for when you arrive at your destination. If you can, book accommodations with cooking facilities to prepare your meals according to your dietary needs. When dining out in unfamiliar places, rely on the research you previously conducted to find suitable restaurants or grocery stores nearby.

7. Stay active:

Remember, staying heart healthy goes beyond just food choices. Incorporate physical activity into your travels by exploring your surroundings on foot or renting bicycles. Take advantage of hotel gyms or swimming pools. It's also essential to get enough rest and manage stress levels while on the road, as a good night's sleep and relaxation contribute to heart health.

Maintaining a heart-healthy diet while dining out and traveling is possible with some planning, smart choices, and a dash of self-control. By doing research, customizing orders, selecting wisely, and controlling portion sizes, you can enjoy delicious meals while safeguarding your heart health. Furthermore, being prepared while traveling and staying active along the way will ensure that your heart remains in good shape even when exploring new places. So, get ready to embark on your next adventure, armed with the knowledge to prioritize your heart and enjoy a culinary journey that nourishes and supports your overall well-being.

Conclusion

In conclusion, adopting a heart-healthy diet is crucial for overall well-being and longevity. A diet that is low in saturated fats, cholesterol, and sodium, while being rich in fruits, vegetables, whole grains, and lean proteins can significantly reduce the risk of cardiovascular diseases. It is important to note that incorporating regular exercise, managing stress levels, and not smoking are equally important factors in maintaining heart health.

By following a heart-healthy diet, individuals can experience various benefits, including improved cholesterol levels, lower blood pressure, increased energy levels, and a reduced risk of heart disease. Moreover, this dietary approach can lead to weight loss and help manage weight, which is crucial in preventing obesity-related conditions.

Furthermore, a heart-healthy diet is not restrictive or dull. There are plenty of delicious and nutritious foods that can be incorporated into meals, making it a sustainable long-term lifestyle choice. It is a matter of making mindful choices and being aware of nutritional content.

In our fast-paced society, it can be challenging to adhere to a heart-healthy diet consistently. However, small changes can go a long way. Making gradual modifications to our diet and incorporating healthy options can gradually improve heart health and overall well-being.

To round up, a heart-healthy diet is

an essential component of a healthy lifestyle. By prioritizing heart-healthy choices and making conscious efforts to improve our eating habits, we can significantly reduce the risk of cardiovascular diseases and improve our quality of life. So let's make the commitment to nourish our hearts with wholesome foods, and reap the rewards of a healthier, more vibrant life.

www.ingramcontent.com/pod-product-compliance
Lightning Source LLC
Chambersburg PA
CBHW070941260726
48661CB00003B/1077